Baby Shower

_____
_____
_____
_____
_____

Name	Gift

Name	Gift

Name	Gift

Name	Gift

Name	Gift

Name	Gift

Name	Gift

Name	Gift

Name	Gift

Name	Gift

www.ingramcontent.com/pod-product-compliance
Lightning Source LLC
LaVergne TN
LVRC100609080526
838200LV00105B/371